SHIATSU FOR INNER HARMONY AND BALANCE

A slice of Japanese tranquillity

Written by Vera Smayan
Translated by Ciaran Traynor

Health and Wellbeing 50MINUTES.com

What is the difference between shiatsu and acupuncture?

Where can I find a shiatsu practitioner?

How can I become a shiatsu practitioner?

SHIATSU FOR INNER HARMONY AND BALANCE

- **Problem**: shiatsu is a real science based on ancient medicine which is becoming more and more popular in the West. What is the best way to approach this complex and fascinating art of massage, and understand how it works? To what extent can we use it in our everyday lives?
- **Aims**: this guide will help you to understand the basic notions of shiatsu and will allow you to learn how to apply simply pressure techniques on parts of the body to increase your well-being. it will also give you some advice to improve your daily life.
- **FAQs**:
  - Is shiatsu a relaxation or therapeutic treatment?
  - Is shiatsu officially recognised as a medical treatment?
  - Can shiatsu have beneficial effects on psychological problems?
  - What is the difference between shiatsu and acupuncture?
  - Where can I find a shiatsu practitioner?
  - How can I become a shiatsu practitioner?

Shiatsu (literally "finger pressure", from the Japanese *shi* – "fingers", "extremities" – and *atsu* – "pressure") is a relaxing and therapeutic massage which originated in Japan. There are several theories regarding the birth of the art of shiatsu. The most common theory is that it is the fusion of the traditional Japanese massage *anma* – which itself came from the Chinese massage *tui na* and arrived in Japan in the 11th century – and Western chiropractic. In Japan, shiatsu has been recognised as an official medical treatment since the 1950s, although it only appeared in the West in the 1960s and 1970s.

Like acupuncture and moxibustion (a relaxation technique which uses heat to stimulate acupuncture points), shiatsu is based on the principles of traditional Chinese medicine. More specifically, shiatsu uses different pressure, stretching, balance and manipulation techniques to work on the meridians, the channels which circulate energy and link all the body's organs and functions together. Pressure is applied primarily with the fingers, but also with the elbows, the forearms, the feet or even the knees of the practitioner.

Shiatsu acts on the primary systems of the body, both on a physical level as well as on an emotional and mental level. The aim is to help the patient to recover by harmonising and strengthening their body's natural ability to heal itself. The treatment, which is administered while the patient is fully clothed and lying down on a mattress or a futon, can be beneficial to all ages, whatever the person's state of health. The patient then experiences a feeling of extreme lightness and profound calm: the body and mind have been rejuvenated.

Shiatsu is particularly effective when it comes to sleeping and posture problems, reproductive dysfunctions and migraines, but it can also have beneficial effects on emotional or psychological problems, such as depression or even certain psychoses.

<u>**Did you know?**</u>

Shiatsu might be even more ancient than we think. Stone needles dating back to 8000 BC were found in China at Neolithic sites, which implies that the principles of energy in traditional Chinese medicine had already been discovered and studied at this time. Consequently, we can suppose that there were treatments using the hands (rudimentary massages) which preceded or even led to the development of this philosophy.

HOW DOES SHIATSU WORK?

THE BASIC PRINCIPLES

Shiatsu is based on a holistic vision which considers that the body and the mind is a whole and works on energy. This energy circulates throughout the body in channels called meridians. These channels have certain points with a particularly high concentration of energy; these are called *tsubo*, literally "places where energy comes together".

An imbalance in the body's organs and systems can be detected in the relevant meridians and their *tsubo*. This imbalance can appear in different forms in the zones of the body which are associated with them, through symptoms like pain, or a change in skin colour or tone of voice, for example. These symptoms represent clear signals that something is wrong with your inner energy, and this problem can become chronic and gradually turn into an illness over time. Through different energising or calming manipulations applied to the meridians, shiatsu helps the person's vital energy to re-establish the balance of the organs or systems which are having problems. The organism therefore rejuvenates itself completely naturally, and the state of discomfort gets better before finally disappearing.

According to traditional holistic approaches, dysfunction of the mind and body is linked to the person's way of life. This therefore means that our way of thinking and outlook on life, our diet, our personal habits and how we interact with our environment have consequences on our bodies.

Therefore, after treating the patient, the shiatsu practitioner will give them advice to improve their health and prevent a possible relapse, because although the treatment itself can re-establish the balance of their energy, this balance can only be maintained if the person changes what caused the discomfort. These recommendations are based on knowledge of the workings of the body and on what can influence the organism. They can include dietary recommendations, more general advice on quality of life and adapted exercises to reinforce the beneficial effects of the treatment. As in all natural treatments from traditional medicine, the person is encouraged to discover the reason for and the meaning of their problems. In this sense, a shiatsu treatment can be a real opportunity to improve your health and quality of life.

> "I had been suffering from panic attacks for two years. My life had been turned completely upside down. One day, a psychologist suggested that I go to a friend of theirs who was a shiatsu practitioner. The result surpassed all my expectations. I slept for 16 hours straight. When I woke up, I felt different. In the days which followed, I began to feel a certain confidence in my body and began to be less afraid of attacks. And that's how I changed the way I look at myself. Little by little, the attacks faded away." (Ann, 36)

DID YOU KNOW?

Shiatsu is often compared to acupuncture, since they are both based on the same principles, particularly when it comes to the treatment of *tsubo*. Nevertheless, these two practices are very different. It would be wrong to view shiatsu as nothing more than the manipulation of predefined points. In a shiatsu massage, *tsubo* are believed to be found throughout the entire body, given that they are an integral manifestation of energy. With this in mind, pressure applied on a point will have an effect on the energy systems of the whole body. As a result, while acupuncture is based on specific points, shiatsu acts on all points of the body. If we consider the very essence of this art – its application through the hands of a practitioner, which implies multiple dimensions (touch, profound communication, and so on) – we can appreciate the incredible therapeutic power that can be achieved during a shiatsu treatment.

DIAGNOSIS IN SHIATSU TREATMENT

Unlike Western medicine where diagnoses are based on the consideration of symptoms, shiatsu takes a holistic, individual approach and is based on a system which combines observation, smell, hearing and touch. This allows an assessment to be made by taking into account the person in their entirety, including their past experiences and the habits linked to their lifestyle. The point of this type of diagnosis is not only to obtain very precise results, but also to obtain information on the inherent causes of the problem and instructions on the measures to take to stop it from getting worse. By following some simple advice, the person has the opportunity to change the aspects of their life which are causing their illness to develop.

Another interesting aspect of shiatsu is its preventive role, which is to say that it allows health problems to be diagnosed in advance, preventing them from turning into more serious illnesses, such as cancer or senile dementia, through simple therapeutic methods. Shiatsu activates the organism's natural ability to treat itself and re-harmonise rather than imposing invasive remedies which do nothing more than solve, sometimes superficially, a problem which is already very real.

To make their diagnosis, a shiatsu practitioner proceeds through several stages:

- **Observation**, the stage during which the practitioner observes the constituent elements of the person (build, weight, size) and the elements linked to their condition (such as the state of their tongue and their eyes, face and skin, as well as their behaviour, movements, smell and voice).
- **Questioning**, which gives them an idea of the patient's lifestyle and diet.
- **Palpation**, which allows them to define the extent and exact source of the imbalance. This diagnosis is based on the study of the person's *hara*, or abdomen, also called the "ocean of energy" by the Japanese.

A LITTLE RELAXING MASSAGE TO GET YOU STARTED

Here is a massage that can be done at any time. Lie or sit down comfortably, then rub your abdomen and lower stomach with your hand in a clockwise motion.

The motion should be quite slow, and the pressure at times slight and others firm. During the exercise, try to breathe evenly and concentrate on your centre and your feelings. This massage relaxes and activates the entire *hara*, particularly the digestion area.

WHAT ARE THE FOUNDATIONS OF SHIATSU?

THE FIVE ELEMENTS AND THE THEORY OF FIVE TRANSFORMATIONS

The notions of yin and yang are the foundations of Chinese philosophy. According to Chinese cosmology, everything begins with the Tao, a shapeless, hazy and disordered element. It contains the qi, a form of energy with two opposing poles, yin (the force of the earth) and yang (the force of the sky), which create our reality. The yin-yang duality is also the basis of the famous Chinese theory of the five movements (Wu Xing), also called the "five elements", which are Wood, Fire, Earth, Metal and Water and which correspond to the five states of energy, meaning five phases of a cycle of transformation. The entire universe, including man, is governed by the movements of this energy.

The Transformation Cycle

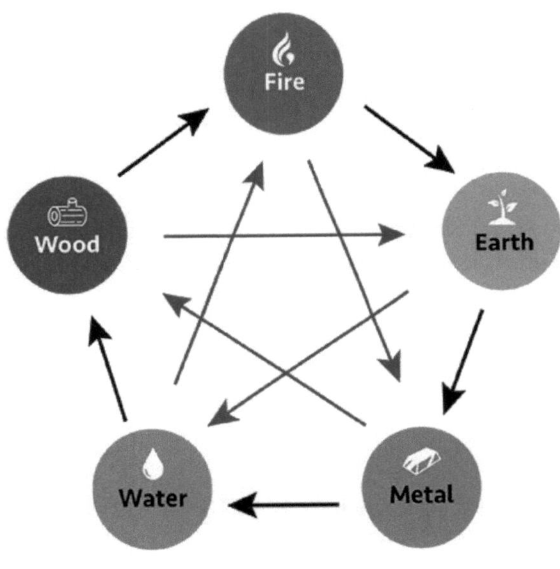

The Generating Cycle
Wood feeds Fire
Fire creates Earth
Earth bears Metal
Metal collects Water
Water nourishes Wood

The Overcoming Cycle
Wood parts Earth
Earth absorbs Water
Water extinguishes Fire
Fire melts Metal
Metal chops Wood

The transformation cycle is a diagram of energy evolution which can be read either as:

- the Sheng cycle, also called the "generating" or "creation" cycle;
- or the Ke cycle, also called the "overcoming" or "destruction" cycle.

Thanks to this diagram and the two laws that govern it, everything in the universe transforms and everything is kept in a constantly renewed state of balance.

This seemingly simple theory is in fact the key to observing the universe. It allows us to establish correspondence between big and small, organs, seasons, directions, tastes, colours, states of the soul, and so on. Every aspect of reality, every phenomenon can be observed and understood thanks to the theory of the Wu Xing movements.

According to traditional Chinese medicine, the organs are subjected to this dynamic of energy transformation. Illness is simply a manifestation of an imbalance in energy, caused by an excess or lack of a particularly element.

TIME FOR SOME SELF-EXAMINATION!

A person's constitution is established from the sum of all their original qualities passed down by their parents and the influence of the diet, activity level and soul of the mother during the nine months of pregnancy. However, it is also influenced by ancestral and environmental factors. A person can be more yang or more yin, depending on the influence of the sky or the earth. Each of these forces is associated with a range of characteristics, and each person possesses special features of both yin and yang; nevertheless, one element will be the dominant one in their structure and expression.

Here is a simple exercise to help you discover your dominant force. Stand in front of a mirror and close your eyes for a few seconds. Breathe deeply and relax. Then, open your eyes and look at yourself. Do you have quite a small build, with thick, light-coloured hair; round, quite small eyes; a little mouth; and a rather square chin? Do you also like physical activity? Are you an extroverted, dynamic, and perhaps sometimes authoritarian person? Then your dominant force is yang. If, on the other hand, you are quite tall and supple, with a round face, rather large eyes and mouth, and a sensitive, emotional personality, then your dominant force is yin.

THE MERIDIANS

The meridians are very closely linked to the theory of yin and yang and that of the five elements, as well as being the basis of traditional Chinese medicine. All of its techniques (acupuncture, moxibustion, acupressure, anma, tai-chi, qi going) are based on the meridians. The theory of the meridians was cited as early as *The Inner Canon of the Yellow Emperor*, the bible of traditional Chinese medicine, the most recent version of which was written in the 1st century BC based on other, more ancient texts.

The meridians are the channels in which the body's vital energy (the qi) circulates in order to nourish all of its tissues and organs. The meridians regulate the harmony and balance of the organism, which behaves as a functional unit.

There are 12 main meridians in the network, all of which are directly linked to one of the five elements and which follow a very specific path. Each pair of meridians (a yin and a yang) is also associated with a colour, a season, a climate, an organ, and so on. Here are two tables summarising the main correspondences for each element.

Element	Wood	Fire	Earth	Metal	Water
Yin-yang phase	Little yang	Big yang	Yin-yang balance	Little yin	Big yin
Energy movement	Mobilisation, exteriorisation	Superficialisation	Distribution	Internalisation	Concentration
Direction	East	South	Centre	West	North
Colours	Green, light blue	Red, orange	Yellow, beige, ochre	White, silver	Black, dark blue
Planet	Jupiter	Mars	Saturn	Venus	Mercury
Evolution	Birth	Growth	Maturity	Old age	Death
Season	Spring	Summer	Transition	Autumn	Winter
Climate	Windy	Hot	Humid	Dry	Cold
Emotions	Anger	Joy, fright, pleasure	Concern, reflexion, worries	Sadness, sorrow	Fear, anxiety

Element	Wood	Fire	Earth	Metal	Water
Tastes	Acidic, sour	Bitter	Sweet, sugary	Spicy, arid	Salty
Smells	Rancid	Burnt	Perfumed	Bitter	Putrid, mouldy
Organs	Liver	Heart	Spleen, pancreas	Lung	Kidney
Senses	Sight	Taste	Touch	Smell	Sound
Tissue and others	Tendons, nails, complexion, limbs	Blood vessels	Muscles, lips, flesh, cells	Skin, body hair, teeth, breasts	Bones, marrow, hair, genitalia, immune system
Body fluid	Tears	Sweat	Saliva	Mucus	Urine

As you can see, Water is associated with the Kidney (yin) and Bladder (yang) Meridians, the colour black, winter, putrid smells, salty foods and the cold.

TIME FOR SOME SELF-EXAMINATION!

We often express our need to rebalance the energy of one of the five elements through the colours we choose to wear, whether consciously or not. For example, people who often wear white or black are trying to amplify or reduce their Metal or Water energy, respectively.

Do you feel the need to dress yourself in a particularly colour? Which colour? Have a look at the table to find out what this colour corresponds to. Then study the other associations it has, such as the organ, season or emotion. The result may surprise you.

THE CIRCADIAN RHYTHM

The qi circulates in the body according to a circadian rhythm, going from one meridian to another. One meridian therefore becomes more active than the others for two hours when its function is essential for the organism.

The circadian rhythm

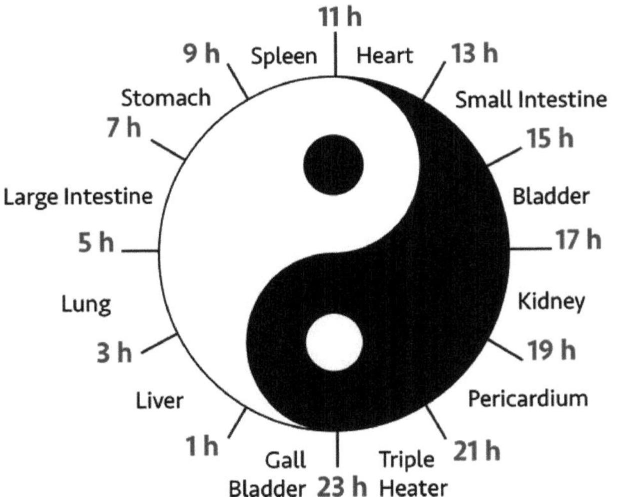

As you can see, the Lung is most active between three and five o'clock in the morning, while the Stomach meridian reaches its most active point between seven and nine o'clock in the morning.

The period when each meridian is most active gives important indications for the diagnosis and, consequently, for the treatment.

TIME FOR SOME SELF-EXAMINATION!

Take a bit of time for yourself to relax and think about your daily life. Are there moments during the day where you feel more tired or more worked up? Is there a recurring phenomenon in your life which appears at more or less the same time almost every day? Note all of these details down and compare them to the meridian circadian rhythm table. You may find out some valuable information about the origin of the problem. For example, if you regularly suffer from insomnia and cannot sleep between one o'clock and three o'clock in the morning, it is possible that you are suffering from an imbalance in your Liver energy.

Thinking about the circadian rhythm of your meridians will also allow you to think about your lifestyle and see how to adapt it to experience each moment in harmony with the natural function that it is associated with.

WHAT IS YOUR ENERGY STATE?

Unlike your constitution, your energy condition is constantly changing because it is the result of your everyday life. By observing your appearance and your behaviour, it is possible to understand the state of your health and improve it by balancing your lifestyle.

Before going any further, try a little exercise. Sit yourself down comfortably and close your eyes for a few seconds. Breathe deeply and relax. Then, open your eyes and think about your current condition. Which emotion is dominating your life at the moment? How would you describe your smell? Which taste is most attractive to you at the moment? Now compare these details with the table of the elements and their associations, and find the element which coincides with your condition. If, for example, you are often sad, you would say your smell is rather acrid and you feel the need to eat spicy foods, then the element you are looking for is Metal.

Read the next chapter for a small section on all the elements and their associations. You will find useful indications on your condition and points which you can treat to improve your energy state.

SHIATSU IN PRACTICE

Now that you have identified the origin(s) of your unbalanced energy, you will learn more about the foundations of shiatsu. In this chapter, you will find a brief description of the five elements, as well as general information on the characteristics associated with each of them and on the meridians and their symptoms of imbalance. You will also learn several pressure points.

METAL

Description

The Metal Table

Direction	West
Colours	White, silver
Season	Autumn
Climate	Dry
Emotions	Sadness, sorrow
Taste	Spicy
Smell	Acrid
Sense	Smell

This table corresponds to autumn and the falling of leaves, which turn into humus and feed the earth and its plants. It symbolises purity and interaction with the outside world.

The meridians associated with Metal are those of the Large Intestine (the yang meridian) and the Lung (the yin meridian): the two organs which link the inside of the body to the outside.

A person with balanced Metal energy is well-organised, efficient, positive and good at considering different points of view. However, a person with unbalanced Metal energy will be rigid, inexpressive, withdrawn and speak in a monotone.

Metal energy is associated with the endocrine system, memory, and all the things that the body does automatically, such as breathing.

Symptoms

When your Metal energy is unbalanced, you may suffer from:

- red, puffy or, on the contrary, sunken cheeks,
- swollen lips,
- a cough, puffy eyes, and feel that you have a cold,
- cold hands and feet,
- a tendency to lean forwards slightly,
- feelings of depression and tiredness,
- a tendency to withdraw into yourself,
- hair loss,
- diarrhoea or, on the contrary, constipation,
- skin problems (boils).

The Lung Meridian (Lg) and its main points

The Lung Meridian

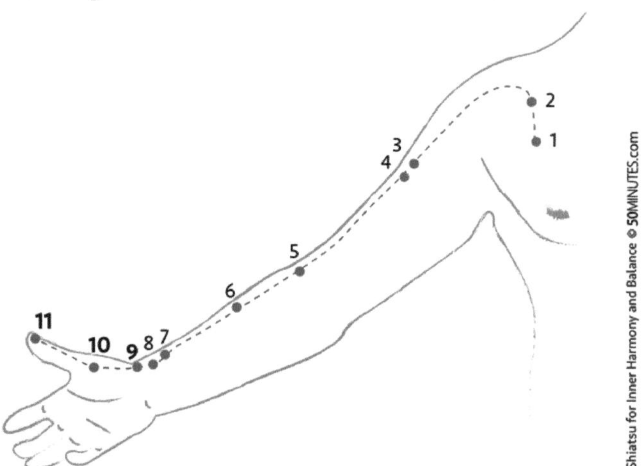

The Lung Meridian is made up of a series of points, with 11 in total.

The **Lg 9 point** is on the inside of the wrist, just where the crease is. It is the place where the pulse can be felt. It is an important point for treating bronchitis and pharyngitis, reducing irritability and strengthening the lungs.

The **Lg 10 point** is found on the side of the palm, in the middle of the first metacarpal bone, where the skin can change colour. Pressure on this point can have positive effects on sore throats, fever, palpitations and emotional suffering.

The **Lg 11 point** is on the radial side of the thumb, at the base of the nail. This point is used for the treatment of tonsillitis, colds, coughs and throat infections. It also has a positive effect on tuberculosis.

TIME FOR SOME SELF-EXAMINATION!

Your shoulders are a powerful indication of the condition of your lungs. People with hunched, sagging shoulders have a yin imbalance in their lungs, which can lead to depression, tiredness, apathy and loss of interest in life. Those with stiff, high shoulders, on the other hand, have a yang imbalance in their lungs, which means they tend to put up walls around themselves and are constantly on the defensive.

The Large Intestine Meridian (LI) and its main points

The Large Intestine Meridian

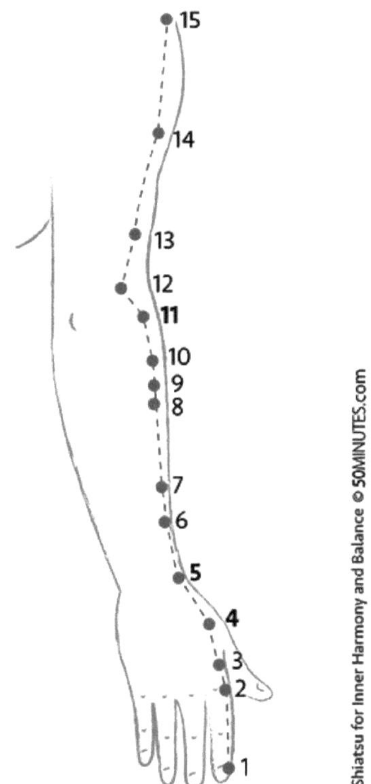

The Large Intestine Meridian is made up of 20 points.

The **LI 4 point** can be found on the back of the hand, at the angle between the first and second metacarpal bones. It is an important point for the recirculation of stagnant energy. It can be used to treat neurasthenia (mental and physical exhaustion), deafness, toothache, atopic dermatitis (an inflammatory, itchy skin disorder), headaches and constipation.

The **LI 5 point** is located between the extensor pollicis longus and brevis tendons. It is used to treat coughs, fever, spasms and tinnitus.

The **LI 11 point** can be found on the protuberance of the supinator muscle and the extensor carpi radialis longus muscle. This is an extremely important point, because it can be used to treat a whole range of skin problems (rosacea, urticaria, eczema, psoriasis) as well as schizophrenia, toothache, amenorrhoea (absence of a menstrual period), and asthenia (general fatigue) if the patient tends to nod off.

EARTH

Description

The Earth Table

Direction	Centre
Colours	Yellow, beige, ochre
Season	Transition
Climate	Humid
Emotions	Concern, reflexion, worries
Tastes	Sweet, sugary
Smell	Perfumed
Sense	Touch

Earth does not correspond to any particular season, but to the period of transition. It is the energy which is traditionally considered to be the centre of the other energies. It represents the return to the centre (to the self) and renewal.

Earth is associated with the Spleen/Pancreas (yin) and the Stomach (yang) Meridians.

Earth energy implies a pragmatic solidity, a good relationship with food and your mother, a good muscle tone, a high intellectual capacity (to reflect, analyse and learn), as well as a tendency to listen to and help others. People with unbalanced Earth energy are anxious, unstable, cannot concentrate on tasks and are too open to others (to the point of wearing themselves out).

Earth redistributes energy with the turning of each season (Spleen/Pancreas), regulates the body's nutritional cycle, governs blood production and the female hormonal system, and keeps liquids in circulation and organs in place.

Symptoms

When your Earth energy is unbalanced, you may suffer from:

- a lilting voice,
- cracked lips,
- cracked hands and heels,
- diarrhoea or constipation,
- problems with digestion or hyperacidity,
- stiff neck and shoulders,
- lack of strength, a feeling of weakness,
- a feeling of cold in the lower part of the body (legs and stomach),
- painful periods,
- obsessions and a tendency to dwell on the negative things in life,
- weight gain or loss.

The Spleen/Pancreas Meridian and its main points

The Spleen/Pancreas Meridian

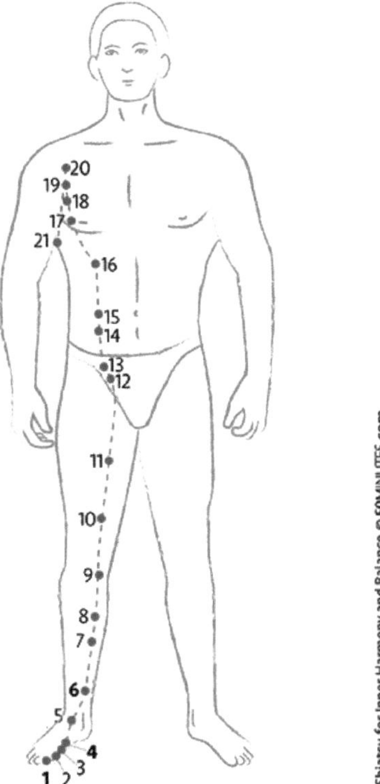

The Spleen/Pancreas Meridian is made up of 21 points.

The **SP 1 point** is found at the inside corner of the big toenail. It is linked with mental illnesses, digestion and stomach pains.

The **SP 4 point** can be found in the middle of the inner side of the first metatarsal bone, at the level of the hollow. It balances the digestion process. It has an influence on appetite problems and on high blood pressure.

The **SP 6 point** can be found four inches above the most protruding part of the inner malleolus, along the tibia bone, between the bone and the tendon. It is the meeting point of three yin meridians, which makes it a very important point. It has a beneficial effect on period pain and insomnia. It rebalances blood production and encourages its circulation in the lower limbs. Make sure not to stimulate this point too much if you are pregnant, as it may lead to a miscarriage.

The Stomach Meridian (S) and its main points

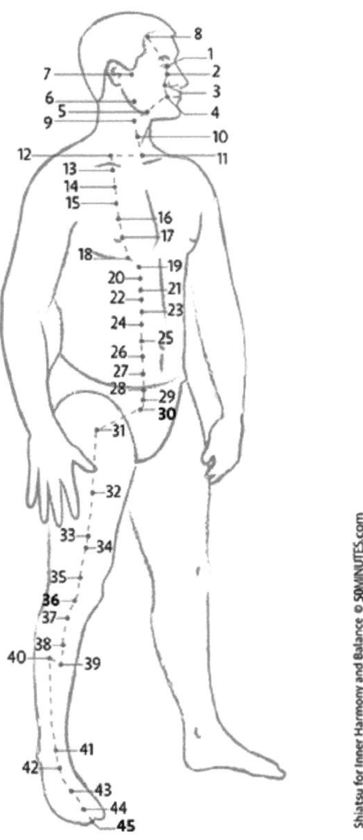

The Stomach Meridian is made up of 45 points.

The **S 30 point** is located on the lower abdomen, two or three inches below the belly button. It encourages blood circulation and has a positive effect on digestive problems and gynaecological diseases.

The **S 36 point** is found on the knee, about an inch below the depression formed by the kneecap and the ligament. It plays a role in the general tone of the body and has a beneficial effect on problems with the nervous system, nausea and lack of appetite.

The **S 45 point** can be found on the outer side of the base of the second toenail. It regulates appetite and can be used to treat asthenia.

WATCH OUT!

An unbalanced Earth energy can also be detected by constantly singing or humming, even when you are not aware that you are doing it! To put this energy back into balance, begin by cutting down on sugary foods, including fruits, and increasing your consumption of wholegrains.

FIRE

Description

The Fire Table

Direction	South
Colours	Red, orange
Season	Summer
Climate	Hot
Emotions	Joy, fright, pleasure
Taste	Bitter
Smell	Burned
Sense	Taste

The Fire element corresponds to heat and summer. It is the most dynamic state of energy, capable of spreading quickly throughout the body and able to illuminate, heat, stimulate and overheat. It is closely linked with emotions and with the ability to be in harmony with others.

The Heart (yin) and Small Intestine (yang) Meridians are associated with Fire, as are the Pericardium (yin) and the Triple Heater (yang) Meridians. These last two are not associated with a particular organ, but with a function. They both have a broader role to play. The Pericardium and the Triple Heater control and balance the Heart and the Small Intestine's relationships with all the other organs. The role of the Pericardium is to transmit the heart's orders to the rest of the body; it is the "minister" in charge of relaying and harmonising everything that happens in the body in relation to the heart. As for the Triple Heater, its job is to ensure communication between the body's large organs, thereby balancing the breathing, digestion and elimination systems.

A harmonious Fire energy can be seen through an ability to get on well with people, enjoyment in life, an ability to adapt easily, a balanced mental and emotional state, spirituality, self-confidence and charisma. On the other hand, an unbalanced Fire energy will lead to hyperexcitation, sudden changes in interest, muddled thoughts, possessiveness and greed.

Fire links a person's spiritual side to their material side and controls emotions, blood circulation and mental balance.

Symptoms

When your Fire energy is unbalanced, you may suffer from:

- a red or swollen nose tip,
- red or very white skin around the cheekbones,
- circulation problems,
- bright eyes,
- speech problems (mental blocks and aphasia),
- extreme sweating and hot flushes,
- ear problems,

- the feeling of having a weight around your solar plexus,
- violent behaviour,
- schizophrenia.

The Lower Intestine (LI) Meridian and its main points

The Small Intestine Meridian

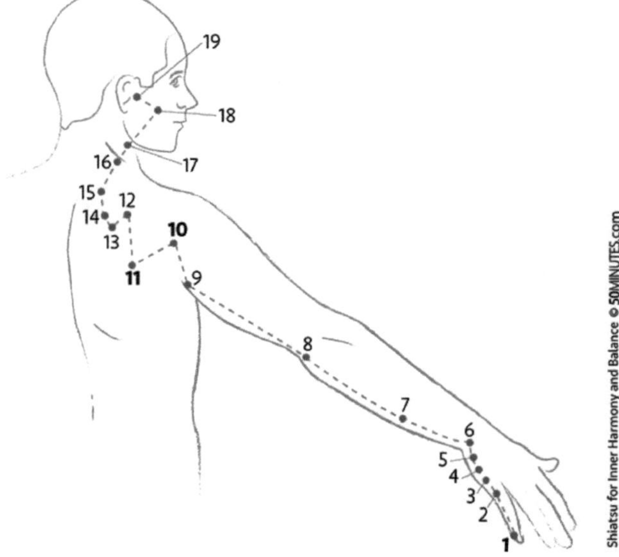

The Lower Intestine Meridian has 19 points.

The **LI 1 point** is at the base of the inner nail of the little finger. It can help with fainting fits, intercostal cramps, sore throats and headaches.

The **LI 10 point** can be found in the fold of the upper arm, in the hollow which forms when the arm is raised. It can help shoulder and elbow problems as well as shoulder and neck stiffness.

The **LI 11 point** is found in the centre of the armpit. It can relieve shoulder and chest pain as well as neuralgia.

The Heart Meridian (H) and its main points

The Heart Meridian

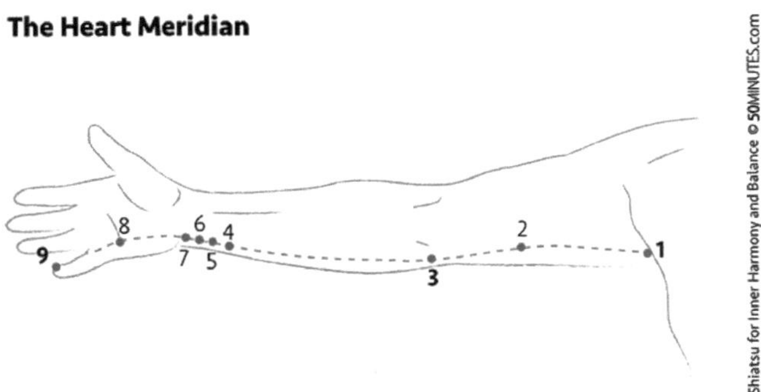

The Heart Meridian is made up of 9 points.

The H 1 point can be found in the hollow of the armpit. It can relieve insomnia, night sweats and have a beneficial effect on certain voice problems.

The H 3 point is located at the end of the ulna (a long bone which stretches from the elbow to the fingers) at the joint between the elbow bend and the entepicondyle (the bony projection of the humerus bone in the upper arm). It can be useful in the treatment of stress and hyperarousal, and can also be used to ease palpitations.

The H 9 point is located on the outer part of the nail of the little finger. It is an invigoration point of the heart.

The Pericardium Meridian (P) and its main points

The Pericardium Meridian

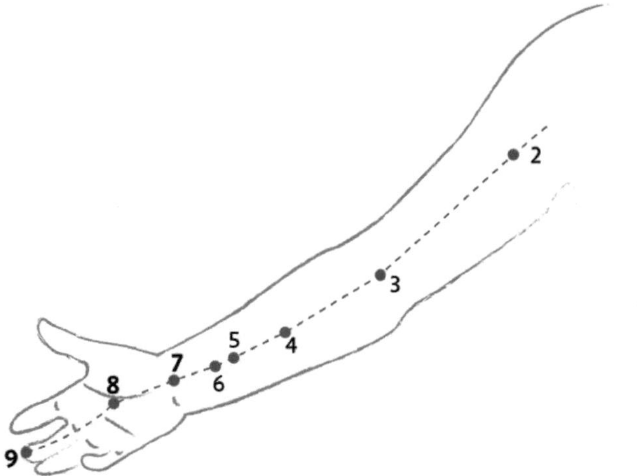

The Pericardium Meridian is made up of 9 points.

The **P 7 point** is in the centre of the wrist, between the two flexor carpi radialis muscles. It can alleviate vomiting. It is also a very important resuscitation point.

The **P 8 point** can be found in the middle of the palm, at the point the middle finger touches when it is bent. It is used to treat restlessness, palpitations and tachycardia.

The **P 9 point** is located at the end of the middle finger, near the nail. It is a very important invigoration point. It can be used to treat fatigue and insomnia.

The Triple Heater (TH) Meridian and its main points

The Triple Heater Meridian

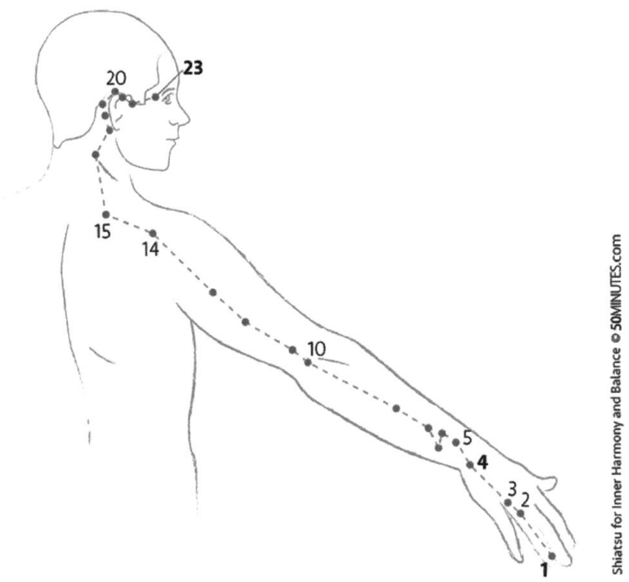

The Triple Heater Meridian is made up of 23 points.

The **TH 1 point** can be found in the inner corner of the ring fingernail. It can be used to treat fevers, the flu, urticaria and eczema.

The **TH 4 point** is located on the back of the wrist, in the hollow of the ulna. It is helpful in treating dyspepsia, aerophagia and tinnitus, and can also have a positive effect on neck stiffness.

The **TR 23 point** is at the end of the eyebrow. It has positive effects on eye problems, migraines and facial neuralgia.

WATER

Description

The Water Table 💧

Direction	North
Colours	Black, dark blue
Season	Winter
Climate	Cold
Emotions	Fear, anxiety
Taste	Salty
Smells	Putrid, mouldy
Sense	Hearing

Water corresponds to winter and represents the transitional state of deep sleep before the beginning of a new cycle. It is therefore the element associated with restoration, regeneration and reflexion. It is a type of fluctuating energy with two sides to it: it is calm and clear while still being very deep and powerful, almost threatening.

This energy is linked to the Bladder (yang) and Kidney (yin) Meridians and has a role of dissolution, just like its element. It is a form of basic energy (which can be found in the kidneys), and is therefore a part of a person's constitution. It governs the bones, joints, spinal cord, brain, hair, kidneys bodily fluids (urine), reproductive organs and adrenal glands.

A person with a balanced Water energy is brave, takes initiative, adapts easily and deals with stress well. They find it easy to communicate with others, particularly with their family. They are sensitive, reach their goals, have a sense of moderation, enjoy a solid constitution and are in good health. However, if their Water energy is out of sync, they will be timid, skittish, introverted, unsure of themselves and often very condescending.

Symptoms

When your Water element is out of balance, you may experience:

- thin hair which breaks easily,
- extreme fatigue,
- hot flushes,
- swollen legs,
- shivers,
- the feeling that your thoughts are muddled,
- migraines,
- general tension,

- uterus dysfunction.

The Kidney (K) Meridian and its main points

The Kidney Meridian

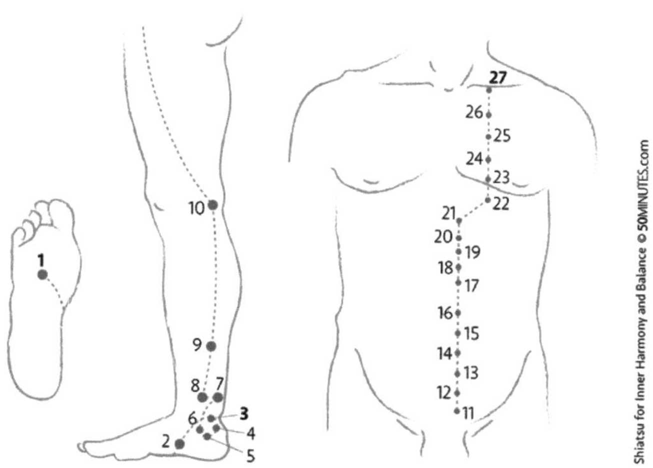

The Kidney Meridian is made up of 27 points.

The **K 1 point** can be found on the sole of the foot, in the hollow between the second and third metatarsals. It is an important resuscitation point. It is also used to treat kidney problems and can help to calm agitated and worried minds.

The **K 3 point** is found in the hollow behind the internal malleolus (inner side of the ankle) at its most prominent part, in front of the Achilles tendon. It is an important energy invigoration point. It is also necessary in the treatment of kidney problems and rheumatism. Finally, it can be used to treat back pain.

The **K 27 point** is found at the angle of the collar bone, sternum and the first rib bone. It disperses excess energy throughout the body.

The Bladder (B) Meridian and its main points

The Bladder Meridian

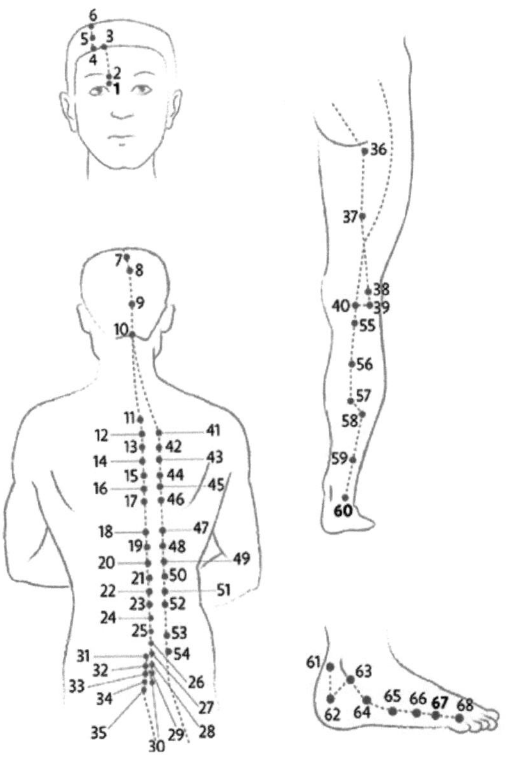

The Bladder Meridian is made up of 68 points.

The **B 1 point** can be found above the inner corner of the eye. It is used to treat sinusitis, brain fatigue, and eye and vision problems.

The **B 60 point** can be found behind the internal malleolus, but before the Achilles tendon. It is used to combat diarrhoea, menstrual pain and cystitis. It also useful in the treatment of neck and head pain.

The **B 67** is located at the corner of the fourth toenail. It regulates the energy in the lower body, heals migraines and contributes to general relaxation. However, make sure not to stimulate this point too much if you are pregnant, as it may lead to a miscarriage.

WOOD

Description

The Wood Table

Direction	East
Colours	Green, light blue
Season	Spring
Climate	Windy
Emotion	Anger
Tastes	Acidic, sour
Smell	Rancid
Sense	Sight

Wood represents plants, spring, birth, beginnings and growth. It is therefore the energy of creation and continuous change, which presents a great degree of flexibility and adaptation.

This element is associated with the Liver (yin) and Gaul Bladder (yang) Meridians.

A person with balanced Wood energy is creative, lively, flexible and tolerant. They have the ability to plan and make decisions. They are also very moral. An unbalanced Wood element can lead to irritability, outbursts of anger, occasionally excessive responses or emotions, a very authoritarian temperament, a feeling of instability, and mental and emotional confusion.

YOUR TURN!

Wood energy is associated with the spring and is responsible for the detox of the organism. Therefore, at the beginning of spring, try to invigorate your Wood energy by setting yourself a two-week diet based on a high consumption of green vegetables and vegetable sprouts, light soups and steamed fish or white meat.

Symptoms

When your Wood element is out of balance, you may experience:

- a feeling of paralysis (obstructions),
- stiff muscles,
- coordination problems,
- anger or depression,
- a skewed view of reality,
- joint problems and arthritis,
- brittle nails,
- migraines,
- haemorrhoids or prostate pain,
- urticaria.

The Gall Bladder (GB) Meridian and its main points

The Gall Bladder Meridian

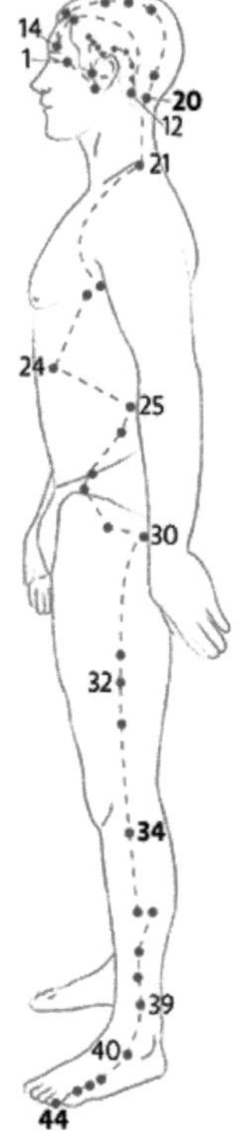

The Gall Bladder Meridian is made up of 44 points.

The **GB 20 point** is located in the depression of the trapezius and sternocleidomastoid muscles. It is an invigoration point which is used in the treatment of eye and ear problems. It is also used to alleviate vertigo and high blood pressure.

The **GB 34 point** is located in the hole below and in front of the lower extremity of the femur. It is effective in the treatment of muscle problems and sprains. It can also be used to cure constipation. It is advisable to treat this point at the turn of each season.

The **GB 44 point** can be found in the corner of the fourth toenail. It is used to treat asthma, agitation and uterus dysfunction.

The Liver (Lr) Meridian and its main points

The Liver Meridian

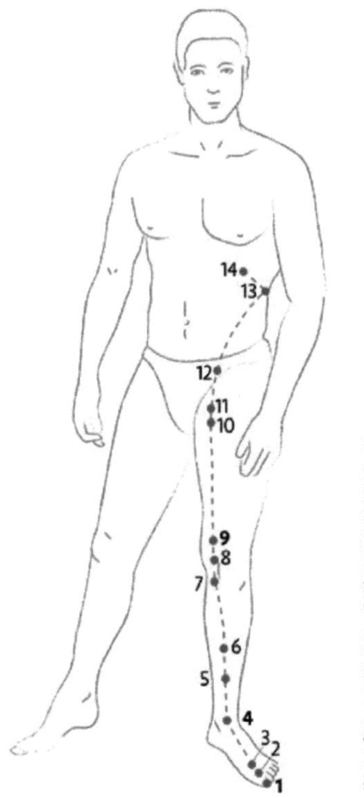

The **Lr 1 point** can be found at the edge of the big toenail, in the middle. It governs the regularisation of the meridian and menstrual cycles. It is also effective in the treatment of migraines, vomiting and spasms.

The **Lr 4 point** can be found on the sole of the foot, between the tendons. It is an invigoration point. It can be used to resolve eye and urogenital problems. It also calms muscle pain.

The **Lr 9 point** is located on the inner thigh, around five inches above the knee, in the hollow between the muscles. It is a very important point in the treatment of uterus dysfunction. It allows you to calm menstrual pain and regulate your cycle. It can also be used to treat impotence.

SHIATSU AND WELLBEING: SOME ADVICE TO LIVE A BETTER LIFE

EVERYTHING COMES BACK TO RELAXATION

Our body's ability to rebalance itself is directly linked to our ability to relax. Why?

The nervous system is made up of two parts, the voluntary nervous system and the autonomic nervous system. The autonomic nervous system is made up of two branches: the parasympathetic nervous system and the sympathetic nervous system, which work together to keep us in balance with our environment. The sympathetic nervous system acts like a protection system: it evaluates and controls external stimuli until the parasympathetic system adapts to them. Prolonged overstimulation of these defences can lead to illnesses.

In our modern society, there is a multitude of stimuli which can chronically overload our sympathetic system and thereby weaken our parasympathetic system. Traffic, lights, phone vibrations, electronic devices, Wi-Fi signals and so on all lead to the chronic overstimulation of the adrenal glands (the glands which are responsible for stress management), accelerating heart rate and digestion problems. The sympathetic system becomes hyperactive, which causes stress and depression, while the parasympathetic system grows weaker and weaker.

Shiatsu can regulate the situation since it can profoundly

stimulate the parasympathetic system, thereby rebalancing the sympathetic system. These changes affect all levels of being, from the physical to the spiritual.

In the period following shiatsu treatment, patients naturally begin to search for new paths to improve their wellbeing, paying more attention to their diet and physical condition, and will be more open to other forms of therapy.

THE KEYS TO A NEW YOU

Breathing

All relaxation and meditation practices include breathing techniques. Deep breathing stimulates oxygenation – and therefore also stimulates the parasympathetic system – and regulates the sympathetic nervous system.

How does it do this? Stable, regular breathing facilitates the absorption of oxygen, allows you to expel carbon dioxide and directly influences the nervous system, while weak, irregular breathing creates a build-up of carbon dioxide in the body, and therefore increases the acidity of the blood, which in turn creates a state of stress. Good breathing is therefore essential.

A LITTLE RELAXING EXERCISE

Sit on the ground, close your eyes and relax. Take a slow, deep breath through your nose, filling first your lungs and then your stomach with air, concentrating your attention on the area around your belly button. It is important that your stomach swell. Hold your breath and count to five. Next, slowly breathe out through your nose, emptying your lungs and pressing down on your stomach to expel all of the air. Repeat this exercise at least three times. You will feel calmer and your body will be re-oxygenated. You can repeat this exercise at any time during the day.

Diet

Diet is the key to maintaining balance in the body and the mind. Today, our diet is often based on heavy animal products and is high in refined, saturated fat, which has a negative impact on our health. A macrobiotic diet is the first step towards a real existential change.

THE MACROBIOTIC DIET

The macrobiotic diet (from the Greek *makros*, "long", and *bios*, "life") is not only a list of dietary rules to follow, but also a philosophy of life based on the Eastern theory of yin and yang. The aim of the macrobiotic diet is to achieve a balance between these two forces. The best way to do that is to eat yin foods (grains, peas, and courgettes, for example) with yang foods (carrots, goats' cheese, and potatoes, for example).

Refined foods create acidity in the body, while whole foods are in harmony with our digestive system. Cereals and legumes, particular those made from fermented soya, supply the body with easily digestible protein to reconstruct our cells and tissues. Unlike meat, they leave no toxic residue in the organism.

You should therefore try to eat non-refined, preferably organic foods, reduce your meat consumption, and introduce seaweed, which is an extraordinary source of minerals, into your diet.

The Makko Ho energy exercises

There are many disciplines which aim to rebalance our energy state. The most well-known are obviously taichi, qi gong and yoga. However, the exercises most linked to shiatsu are undoubtedly the six base Makko Ho exercises, a series of specific exercises which aim to invigorate the twelve main meridians and improve circulation. The positions are not difficult and can be done by anyone.

The six Makko Ho exercises

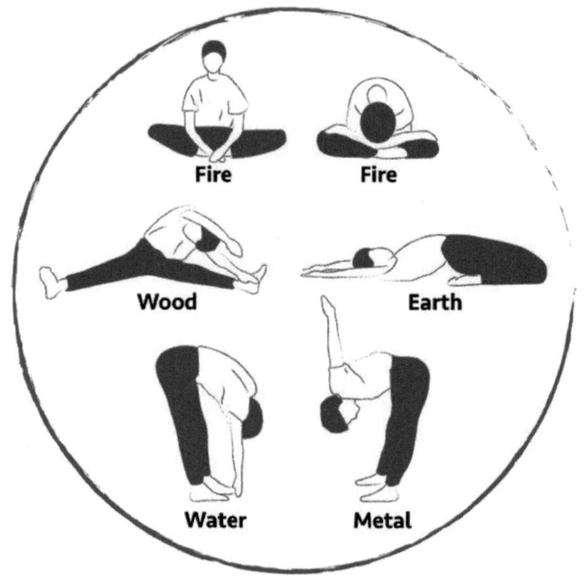

Doing these exercises does not take much time out of your everyday life, but allows you to rebalance your energy system naturally, restore your energy and live better.

The do-in

A self-massage technique based on the principles of traditional Chinese medicine, the do-in can be done alone or in a group, at any point of the day, and can be easily learned with the help of manuals or videos on the internet. These massages allow you to invigorate and rebalance the energy of the twelve meridians through tapping, finger pressure on the *tsubo* and rubbing.

A LITTLE DO-IN HAND MASSAGE

This do-in massage can be done at any time of the day, even at the office. Begin by rubbing your hands on both sides, as if you are trying to clean them. Then, make circular motions with your wrists. Next, take each finger in turn with your other hand. Rub each one at the base of the nail, then press down on the two sides, pulling slightly outwards. After this, rub the palm of your hand from the middle to the edges, then press on the centre of your palm, where your fingers rest when they are bent, and then on the point located in the hollow between the first and second metacarpal bones. Finish the exercise by shaking your hands, with your fingers pointing towards the floor.

FAQS

IS SHIATSU A RELAXATION OR THERAPEUTIC TREATMENT?

Shiatsu is both a relaxation and a therapeutic treatment. The two go hand in hand, because our physical functioning and our ability to rebalance ourselves are linked to our ability to relax.

Shiatsu deeply stimulates the parasympathetic system, which is usually weakened, and creates balance in the sympathetic system, which is often overstimulated. As a result, the causes of stress are diminished. In doing so, the development of illnesses is also slowed.

IS SHIATSU OFFICIALLY RECOGNISED AS A MEDICAL TREATMENT?

Shiatsu has been officially recognised as a medical treatment in Japan since 1955. However, it was only recognised in the West later on, and only by a certain number of states and health organisations. The European Parliament accepted it as alternative medicine in 1997 (*Report on the status of non-conventional medicines*). In Europe, there is a shiatsu organisation called the European Shiatsu Federation (ESF), which certifies shiatsu teaching at different schools and provides a list of qualified practitioners.

CAN SHIATSU HAVE BENEFICIAL EFFECTS ON PSYCHOLOGICAL PROBLEMS?

Shiatsu is based on a holistic view which considers the body and the mind as two parts of a whole. As a result, a physical problem will have behavioural or emotional consequences. By acting on energy, shiatsu has a simultaneous effect on every level and allows the patient to feel better in body and mind.

WHAT IS THE DIFFERENCE BETWEEN SHIATSU AND ACUPUNCTURE?

Shiatsu and acupuncture are two techniques with their origins in traditional Chinese medicine. Both are based on energy principles from Chinese philosophy, particularly the existence of energy (qi) which circulates through channels called meridians, where it is concentrated on points called *tsubo*. The major difference lies in the nature of the two techniques.

Acupuncture treats *tsubo* through needles, locating them with precision and associating them with a series of factors (the time of day, the season, and so on).

In shiatsu, every part of the body is important. Since shiatsu is a massage technique which also includes stretches and manipulations, practitioners can act on several parts of the body at the same time.

WHERE CAN I FIND A SHIATSU PRACTITIONER?

The easiest way to find a shiatsu practitioner is to contact the <u>European Shiatsu Federation</u>. They can give you a list of approved shiatsu practitioners.

HOW CAN I BECOME A SHIATSU PRACTITIONER?

There are several schools approved by the European Shiatsu Federation which organise professional classes. Training to be a practitioner takes three years. At the end of this period, after sitting various exams and having carried out a certain amount of treatments organised by the school, the practitioner-in-training has to sit an entrance exam for the ESF. Consult the <u>organisation's page</u> for more information.

We want to hear from you!
Leave a comment on your online library
and share your favourite books on social media!

FURTHER READING

BIBLIOGRAPHY

- Goodman, S. (2004) *Manuel de praticien*. Paris: Éditions Trédaniel.
- Kushi, M. (2009) *Le livre de la macrobiotique*. Paris: Éditions Trédaniel.
- Kushi, M. (2009) *Le livre du diagnostic oriental*. Paris: Éditions Trédaniel.
- Masunaga, S. (1985) *Zen shiatsu, comment équilibrer le yin et le yang pour une meilleure santé*. Paris: Éditions Trédaniel.
- Masunaga, S. (1985) *Zen shiatsu, exercices visualisés : Travail des méridiens pour le bien-être*. Paris: Éditions Trédaniel.
- Namikoshi, T. (2004) *Le livre complet de la thérapie shiatsu*. Paris: Éditions Trédaniel.

ADDITIONAL SOURCES

- Jarmey, C. and Mojay, G. (1999) *Shiatsu, Revised Edition: The Complete Guide*. London: Thorsons.
- Liechti, E. (2016) *The Extended Meridians of Zen Shiatsu*. London: Singing Dragon.

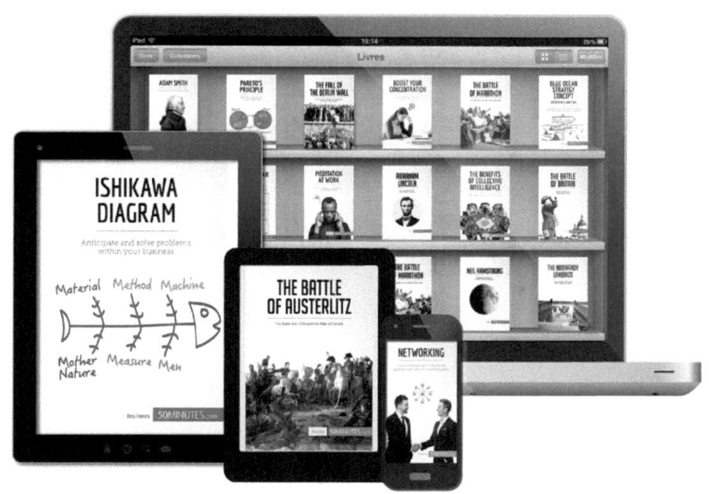

IMPROVE YOUR GENERAL KNOWLEDGE

IN A BLINK OF AN EYE !

www.50minutes.com

www.50minutes.com

Ebook EAN: 9782808001724

Paperback EAN: 9782808001731

Legal Deposit: D/2017/12603/606

Cover: © Primento

Digital conception by Primento, the digital partner of publishers.